Alaska Pox 2024

From Mystery to Mastery - Charting the Course for Prevention and Protection

Brian A. Godfrey

TABLE OF CONTENTS

INTRODUCTION

What is Alaska Pox?

Imagine a virus wrapped in mystery, developing stealthily amid the vast Alaskan tundra. This is the story of Alaska Pox, a recently discovered orthopoxvirus that has aroused the imagination of experts and the public alike. While it is currently rare, knowing its nature and possible consequences is vital. So, let's begin on a voyage to expose the mysteries of Alaska Pox, answering the questions that could be churning in your mind:

1. A Newcomer on the Viral Scene
Discovered in 2015, Alaska Pox belongs to the same family as infamous viruses like smallpox and monkeypox. However, fear not, since it carries substantial differences. Unlike its famed siblings, Alaska Pox mostly affects tiny animals like voles and shrews,

with only a few human cases identified so far.

2. Unveiling the Symptoms
Should you acquire Alaska Pox, what can you expect? The most telltale indication is the development of one or more skin lesions, appearing as lumps or pustules. Think along the lines of bug bites, but maybe bigger and more persistent. Alternative symptoms could include enlarged lymph nodes, joint discomfort, and muscle pains, making it necessary to seek expert evaluation to rule out alternative causes.

3. The Transmission Enigma
How can Alaska Pox transfer from animals to humans? The answer remains a fascinating conundrum. While the particular route of transmission is still under research, experts believe interaction with sick animals or their tissues might play a major role. This underlines the significance of exercising

proper hygiene and avoiding direct contact with wild animals, especially if you work or spend time outside in Alaska.

4. A Spectrum of Severity

Thankfully, most instances of Alaska Pox documented so far have been mild, disappearing within a few weeks without requiring particular treatment. However, it's vital to understand that individual experiences might differ. In rare situations, particularly for people with weak immune systems, the virus can lead to more serious sickness.

5. The Evolving Landscape of Research

The scientific world is aggressively uncovering the secrets of Alaska Pox. Research efforts are focused on understanding its genesis, transmission patterns, possible consequences, and creating diagnostic methods. Studying how the virus interacts with the human immune system is also crucial for determining the necessity of future therapies like vaccinations.

History and discovery of the virus

The Alaskan wilderness, with its beautiful vistas and rich animals, has mysteries yet to be uncovered. Among them lies the story of Alaska Pox, a recently discovered virus that has aroused scientific intrigue and popular attention. While it is currently rare, knowing its historical path and the circumstances surrounding its discovery is vital for future studies and public health initiatives. So, brace up as we continue with a deep investigation of the history and discovery of Alaska Pox:

The Glimmers of the Unknown: 2010-2014

The tale begins in the unspoiled Alaskan wilderness. Unbeknownst to the world, the virus quietly spread amongst tiny animals like voles and shrews, patiently awaiting its day on the scientific stage.

2015: The First Encounter

The tipping point happens in an apparently normal incident. A resident of Fairbanks, Alaska, appears with odd skin lesions and enlarged lymph nodes. Initial diagnoses tend toward common illnesses, but something doesn't quite match.

Enter the Viral Detectives

Enterprising public health professionals and experts suspect something more. Samples are sent for comprehensive examination, beginning on a trip through a maze of diagnostic procedures.

Unraveling the Mystery

Using cutting-edge molecular tools, scientists make a revolutionary discovery. What is the cause behind the strange symptoms? A hitherto discovered orthopoxvirus, separate from its notorious cousins like smallpox and monkeypox. The term "Alaska Pox" is christened, heralding the advent of a new chapter in virology.

Piecing Together the Puzzle
The Early Days
Research moves into high gear. Scientists explore the virus's genetic makeup, discovering its distinctive traits and putting it inside the orthopoxvirus family. Understanding its evolutionary history becomes a focus, seeking to pinpoint its origins and potential animal reservoirs.

The Animal Connection
Studies focus on Alaska's animals, seeking out the virus's native home. The quest leads to tiny animals like voles and shrews, where Alaska Pox is found spreading freely. The jigsaw begins to form a zoonotic virus, migrating from animals to people.

The Transmission Enigma

But how does the leap occur? The specific mechanism of transmission remains an unsolved enigma. Scientists suggest interaction with diseased animals or their tissues as a probable culprit. The significance of excellent hygiene and ethical contact with wildlife becomes clear.

Beyond the First Case

Thankfully, the original episode remained an isolated incident for several years. However, in 2021, six further instances are detected, all within the Fairbanks region. This cluster raises doubts about the virus's potential for human-to-human transfer, necessitating additional inquiry.

The Evolving Narrative
The Present Day:

Research into Alaska Pox continues at a fast pace. Understanding its whole spectrum of virulence, possible problems, and long-term consequences continues to be at the forefront. Additionally, creating diagnostic tools and studying the prospect of future therapies like vaccinations are essential components of ongoing research. Knowledge is Power: While the risk presented by Alaska Pox now looks modest, awareness and education are crucial. Understanding its history, mechanisms of transmission, and individual risk factors helps individuals make educated decisions about their health and relationships with the natural environment.

The Importance of Knowing Alaska Pox

In the immense wilderness of Alaska lies a recently discovered virus termed Alaska Pox, cloaked in mystique and begging the question: Why does it matter? While now posing a small threat, recognizing its relevance extends far beyond immediate concerns. It's an intriguing scientific mystery, a possible public health risk, and a reminder of the interdependence between humans and the natural world. So, let's go on a trip to comprehend the relevance of understanding Alaska Pox.

1. Unveiling the Unknown
Filling the Knowledge Gap:
Alaska Pox is a unique virus, meaning much about its biology, capacity for dissemination, and long-term implications remain unknown. By studying its particular qualities, scientists may address these gaps in information, allowing for improved readiness and informed decision-making.

Unlocking Evolutionary Secrets:
Studying Alaska Pox sheds light on viral evolution, offering significant insights about how new viruses develop and may adapt to diverse settings. This knowledge assists in identifying future dangers and designing wider antiviral solutions.

2. Public Health Implications

Minimizing Risk:
Though currently infrequent, studying Alaska Pox helps assess its potential hazard to public health. Identifying risk factors, transmission mechanisms, and potential problems allows people and communities to take preventative steps and decrease risks.

Preparing for the Future:
Knowledge learned now prepares the way for future readiness. By knowing Alaska Pox today, scientists and public health authorities can build effective response tactics if the virus's behavior changes or its geographical reach extends.

3. Exploring the Human-Animal Interface

Bridging the Divide:
Alaska Pox demonstrates the complex link between humans and animals. Studying its animal reservoirs and transmission patterns gives information on zoonotic illnesses,

influencing measures to reduce human-animal interactions that might encourage viral propagation.

Protecting Ecosystems:
Understanding Alaska Pox's influence on animal populations assists in larger ecosystem conservation efforts. By maintaining wildlife health, we secure our own well-being and the delicate balance of nature.

4. Beyond Alaska
Lessons for Other Emerging Viruses:
The knowledge acquired from researching Alaska Pox can be applied to other developing viruses with zoonotic potential. This greater awareness assists in building general preparedness measures and reaction processes for future threats.

Fueling Scientific Growth:
Research on Alaska Pox leads to the growth of scientific knowledge and technical

instruments. New diagnostic tools, possible vaccinations, and a greater understanding of viral evolution aid not just Alaska Pox research but also the battle against other infectious illnesses.

Part 1: Understanding Alaska Pox

Chapter 1: The Science of Alaska Pox

Classification and characteristics of the virus

Emerging from the vast Alaskan tundra, Alaska Pox provides a compelling scientific enigma. This recently found orthopoxvirus has captivated the attention of experts and the public alike, raising several concerns about its origins, traits, and potential ramifications. Let's begin on a trip to grasp the science underlying Alaska Pox, examining its categorization, distinctive qualities, and the continuous efforts to unravel its intricacies.

Demystifying the Classification

Alaska Pox belongs to the Orthopoxvirus genus, a varied group of viruses infamous for inflicting serious infections, including smallpox and monkeypox. While having many genetic similarities with these famed cousins, Alaska Pox also has distinguishing traits that deserve its own unique categorization. Classified as a species within the Orthopoxvirus genus, it stands apart from its relatives, indicating its distinct evolutionary history.

Peeling Back the Layers: Key Characteristics

Understanding Alaska Pox demands exploring its tiny habitat. Its double-stranded DNA genome, the blueprint for its existence, encodes the machinery required for survival and replication. This genetic coding gives crucial hints about its evolutionary background and prospective behavior. Unlike its near-sibling smallpox, Alaska Pox lacks certain genes linked with virulence, suggesting a milder nature but not removing potential hazards.

Size matters: Compared to other orthopoxviruses, Alaska Pox possesses a smaller genome, a remarkable adaptation presumably connected to its host preferences and ecological niche. Its distinctive envelope protein, the outermost covering of the virus, plays a vital function in detecting and adhering to host cells, perhaps explaining its observed transmission dynamics.

Beyond the Genome: Unveiling Unique Features

The scientific pursuit doesn't end with the genome. Researchers are methodically investigating Alaska Pox's viral particles, the actual form of the virus. Using modern microscopic tools, they are analyzing their structure, form, and surface properties, finding clues about how the virus interacts with host cells and the environment.

Unraveling the Evolutionary Puzzle:

Understanding Alaska Pox's evolutionary history is crucial. Scientists are applying cutting-edge techniques like phylogenetic analysis to trace its genetic origins and identify its closest relatives. This voyage through time gives information on its genesis, probable animal reservoirs, and the evolutionary pressures that molded its distinctive traits.

Host Specificity: A Delicate Balance
Alaska Pox predominantly affects small mammals like voles and shrews, suggesting a degree of host specialization. However, the handful of confirmed human instances raises worries about its capacity to overcome species borders. Researchers are currently exploring the mechanisms controlling this transmission, concentrating on putative zoonotic pathways and environmental impacts.

The Intricate Dance of Replication:
Unlocking the intricacies of Alaska Pox's replication cycle is crucial. Scientists are methodically researching how the virus infects host cells, hijacks their machinery to make more viral particles, and finally bursts forth, possibly infecting other cells. Understanding these complicated

pathways gives significant insights into prospective cures and preventative techniques.

The Quest Continues: Ongoing Research Efforts

The scientific world is aggressively uncovering the mysteries of Alaska Pox. Ongoing research activities focus on:

Developing sophisticated diagnostic tools: Rapid and accurate diagnosis is critical for prompt action and public health monitoring. Researchers are enhancing existing tools and investigating innovative methodologies to identify Alaska Pox infections promptly and effectively.

Understanding transmission dynamics: Pinpointing the specific method of transfer from animals to people remains a critical difficulty. Studies are studying possible pathways, including direct contact, aerosolization, or bites, hoping to inform public health measures and individual risk reduction techniques.

Exploring potential complications: While most recorded occurrences have been minor, recognizing the whole spectrum of possible repercussions is vital. Research is continuing to investigate the possible impact on people with impaired immune systems and find any long-term repercussions.

Vaccine development: Although the current risk is modest, planning is crucial. Researchers are examining the idea of producing vaccinations to prevent future hazards, should the virus's behavior alter or its geographical reach extend.

Looking Beyond the Microscope:
Understanding Alaska Pox spans beyond the technical realm. Researchers are also examining the larger socioeconomic and cultural implications of the virus. Engaging local people, addressing possible fears, and ensuring culturally responsive communication are key parts of ethical research and public health activities.

Genetics and evolution

Emerging from the Alaskan frontier, Alaska Pox has caught the scientific imagination with its unusual genetic composition and compelling evolutionary tale. While it belongs to the legendary Orthopoxvirus genus, a family recognized for producing terrible infections like smallpox and monkeypox,

Alaska Pox exhibits peculiar genetic traits that demand a deeper investigation. Let's begin on a tour through its genetic code, revealing the mysteries of its past and prospective future:

Delving into the Genome:
The heart of Alaska Pox resides inside its double-stranded DNA genome, a blueprint encompassing around 190,000 nucleotides. Compared to its bigger cousins like the variola virus (smallpox), Alaska Pox has a "compacter genome, presumably indicating its adaptation to a different biological niche. This decreased size, however, doesn't translate to simplicity. Its genetic coding includes a plethora of information about its origins, features, and evolutionary journey.

Sequencing the Mystery:
Modern sequencing methods have allowed scientists to sequence the full genome of Alaska Pox, building together a precise genetic map. By comparing this map to other orthopoxviruses, researchers are revealing astonishing insights. While sharing core genes needed for viral replication, Alaska Pox displays unique genetic signatures not observed in its near cousins. These different sequences give evidence regarding its evolutionary route, hinting that possibly an autonomous branch split millions of years ago from a common ancestor.

Genes Tell Tales:
Analyzing particular genes within the Alaska Pox genome gives further, deeper information. Notably, it lacks several genes related to virulence factors seen in

smallpox and monkeypox. This absence signals a potentially milder nature but needs caution: the lack of certain genes doesn't ensure total harmlessness, and study is underway to fully comprehend its virulence potential.

Evolutionary Footprints:
By comparing the Alaska Pox genome to other viruses, scientists may apply a technique called "phylogenetic analysis" to reconstruct its evolutionary history. This approach entails generating a "family tree" based on genetic similarities, allowing researchers to trace the virus's origin and identify its closest cousins. The data show that Alaska Pox separated from other orthopoxviruses roughly 30,000 years ago, likely developing with its chosen small animal hosts in the Arctic and subarctic areas.

Zooming in on Specific Genes:
Several important genes within the Alaska Pox genome warrant specific study. The envelope protein gene encodes the outermost covering of the virus, playing a critical role in identifying and adhering to host cells. Studying this gene helps scientists understand how Alaska Pox infects diverse animals, including possible avenues for zoonotic transmission. Additionally, genes associated with immune evasion are being examined, offering insights into why the virus may occasionally defeat our natural defensive mechanisms.

Beyond the Basics: Exploring Genetic Variation:
The Alaska Pox genome isn't static. Like other living creatures, it can acquire mutations over time, leading to subtle genetic variances within various strains.

Studying this genetic diversity is vital for understanding how the virus could evolve in the future and its capacity to adapt to different habitats or hosts. By identifying these variants, researchers may monitor any changes in virulence or transmission characteristics, allowing for informed public health responses.

Unlocking the Future: Utilizing Genetic Tools

The knowledge acquired from Alaska Pox's DNA is crucial for continuing study and preparation efforts. It supports the development of:

More reliable diagnostic tests: By finding unique genetic sequences peculiar to Alaska Pox, scientists may build tests that promptly and correctly discriminate it from other orthopoxviruses, providing timely diagnosis and proper treatment.

Vaccine development: Understanding the genes involved in viral entrance and immune response lays the road for possible vaccine development. Though the current danger is modest, having a vaccination at hand might prove critical if the virus's behavior changes or its geographical reach extends.
 Antiviral therapies: Studying the viral replication cycle disclosed by the genome helps researchers discover possible targets for antiviral drugs, providing treatment alternatives if needed in the future.

Looking Beyond the Code:
While genetics plays a major part in understanding Alaska Pox, it's essential to remember that evolution is a

complicated interplay between genes and the environment. Studying the ecological niche of Alaska Pox's animal reservoirs, such as voles and shrews, and the probable mechanisms affecting zoonotic transmission are equally crucial components of comprehending its evolutionary route and future hazards.

Animal reservoirs and transmission routes

Alaska Pox provides a captivating scientific puzzle. This recently identified orthopoxvirus, while now offering limited risk, has generated curiosity about its animal reservoirs and how it can transcend the species barrier for humans. By knowing these essential factors, we may better identify possible dangers and adopt effective preventative actions. So, let's continue on a wonderful exploration into Alaska Pox's animal partners and the intriguing paths of its transmission:

The Whispers of the Wild: Identifying Animal Reservoirs

The quest for Alaska Pox's natural habitat brings us deep into the Alaskan ecology. Initial research focused on possible reservoirs among frequently recognized disease carriers, including rats and bats. However, the breakthrough came in 2015, when scientists detected the virus in small mammals, including northern red-backed voles and shrews. Subsequent research verified the occurrence of Alaska Pox in these animals across diverse Alaskan locations, cementing their role as the principal animal reservoirs.

Understanding the Host-Virus Dance:

The link between Alaska Pox and its small animal hosts is an important topic of research. While the virus appears to cause

minimal to no sickness in these animals, it
effortlessly replicates within their cells,
maintaining its life. Studies show a probable
"co-evolutionary history" between Alaska
Pox and its hosts, leading to a balanced
relationship where neither side suffers major
harm.

**Beyond the Obvious: Exploring
Additional Reservoirs:**
While tiny animals presently occupy
attention, experts are studying the idea of
"alternative reservoirs. Factors like probable
regional variances and various animal
populations need a broader strategy.
Studies are exploring additional rodents,
lagomorphs like hares and pikas, and even
predators that could feast on infected small
animals. Understanding the whole spectrum
of possible reservoirs is critical for complete
risk assessment and public health
measures.

The Mystery of Transmission: Unveiling the Pathways:

How does Alaska Pox transcend the gap between animals and humans? This intriguing question remains one of the largest obstacles to understanding the virus. While the specific manner of transmission is still under research, many alternative avenues are being explored:

Direct Contact: Close contact with sick animals or their tissues is a hypothesized route. This includes acts like handling caught animals, skinning hunting animals, or engaging with ill or deceased wildlife.

Indirect Contact: Contamination of the environment with infected animal droppings or secretions might represent a concern, particularly for people working or spending time outside in Alaska.

Aerosols: While the likelihood of airborne transmission requires additional research, it cannot be fully ruled out, especially in poorly ventilated environments or during close contact with diseased animals.

Vectors: The involvement of insects or other animals as vectors conveying the virus from animals to humans remains mostly unknown but demands additional investigation.

Beyond the Alaskan Frontier: Geographic Considerations

Currently, Alaska Pox appears to be largely restricted to the Alaskan ecosystem. However, with increased human mobility and environmental changes, the possibility of its global growth cannot be overlooked. Studying animal migration patterns, examining environmental conditions, and monitoring possible spillovers in nearby regions are critical components of future research and public health preparation.

The Importance of Individual Behavior:
Understanding the various transmission
channels helps individuals make educated
decisions and lower their risk. Practicing
good hygiene, especially after outdoor
activities or possible interaction with wildlife,
is crucial. Avoiding close contact with ill or
dead animals and properly managing
hunting animals are crucial considerations.

**Beyond Individual Actions: Public Health
Interventions**
Public health authorities play a critical role in
reducing the possible spread of Alaska Pox.
This includes:

Surveillance and monitoring: Regularly
monitoring animal populations and human
cases is essential for early detection and
outbreak prevention.

**Public education and awareness
campaigns.** Educating the public about the
virus, its potential transmission routes, and

preventive measures is crucial for responsible behavior and risk reduction. Developing guidelines and regulations: Implementing guidelines for safe handling of wildlife, proper disposal of animal waste, and biosecurity measures in research facilities helps minimize potential spillovers.

Looking Ahead: Future Research Directions

Unraveling the intricacies of Alaska Pox propagation demands continuing study efforts. Key areas of concentration include:

Identifying the dominant mode of transmission: Pinpointing the primary route of transmission from animals to humans is crucial for effective prevention strategies.

Studying viral shedding and persistence in the environment: Understanding how long the virus survives outside its host and potential environmental factors influencing its survival will inform public health interventions.

Investigating the function of viral mutations: Studying how the virus could change and perhaps adapt to different surroundings or hosts is crucial for determining future dangers and readiness.

Chapter 2: Symptoms and Diagnosis

Recognizing the signs and symptoms

Alaska Pox presents a difficulty not only in understanding its origins and transmission but also in swiftly recognizing and treating possible cases. While now offering modest risk, early identification and diagnosis are vital for individual well-being and successful public health initiatives. So, let's begin on a trip to expose the signs and symptoms of Alaska Pox, investigating potential dangers and the instruments available for a correct diagnosis.

The First Clues: Recognizing Symptoms
Unlike its colorful cousins like smallpox, Alaska Pox frequently appears with "milder and perhaps unclear symptoms. However, understanding these telltale indications

allows individuals to seek fast medical treatment and aid in early diagnosis.

The Hallmark Feature: Skin Lesions
The major sign of Alaska Pox is the development of skin lesions. These frequently begin as localized lumps, pustules, or ulcers, first resembling insect bites or other common skin disorders. However, major distinctions exist:

Location: While bug bites generally occur on exposed places like arms and legs, Alaska Pox lesions may grow anywhere on the body, including the palms and soles.

Evolution: Unlike insect bites, which normally heal rapidly, Alaska Pox lesions steadily grow over several weeks, potentially crusting over and leaving scars.

Clustering: While bug bites may look dispersed, Alaska Pox lesions frequently occur in clusters or groups, sometimes following a line where the virus entered the body.

Beyond the Skin: Additional Symptoms
While skin lesions are the defining feature, other symptoms could accompany them, presenting further clues:

Swollen lymph nodes: The lymph nodes nearest to the infected location, for example, in the armpits or groin, may become swollen and painful.

Fever: A slight fever, often low-grade, may be present, especially in the earliest stages of illness.

Muscle aches and joint pain: General aches and pains could develop, albeit typically less severe than in other orthopoxvirus infections.

Fatigue: A general sensation of weariness and malaise is usually described.

The Importance of Individual Experience:
It's crucial to note that individual experiences might differ. Some individuals may only develop modest skin lesions, while others could present with a broader spectrum of symptoms. Additionally, the incubation period, the time between exposure and symptom manifestation, now spans from 5 to 21 days, further underscoring the need for awareness and immediate medical intervention.

Differential diagnosis: Ruling out similar illnesses

Alaska Pox provides difficulty in detecting and treating its modest and often misleading symptoms. While now offering low-risk care, proper and quick diagnosis is vital for individual well-being and successful public health initiatives. So, let's continue on a quest to understand the subtleties of Alaska

Pox symptoms, studying probable lookalikes and the tools available to separate them.

The Masquerade of Symptoms:

Unlike its iconic cousins like smallpox, Alaska Pox frequently wears a mask of modest and sometimes misleading symptoms. While skin lesions remain the signature feature, identifying their subtleties and separating them from comparable illnesses is vital.

The Lookalike Game: Key Differentiators

Several conditions can mimic Alaska Pox, requiring careful comparison and evaluation of particular details.

1. Insect Bites:

Location: Insect bites normally target exposed regions like arms and legs, but Alaska Pox lesions can form anywhere, including palms and soles.

Evolution: Bites heal rapidly, whereas Alaska Pox lesions grow over weeks, potentially crusting and scarring.

Clustering: Bites are dispersed, but Alaska Pox lesions commonly cluster, sometimes following the virus' entrance location. Additional Symptoms: Alaska Pox could manifest with fever, swelling lymph nodes, and malaise, absent in bite responses.

2. Bacterial Skin Infections:
Lesion Appearance: Impetigo and other bacterial illnesses appear with red, weeping lesions, unlike the deeper pustules of Alaska Pox.

Presence of Pus: Bacterial infections generally include yellow or green pus, while Alaska Pox pus is often white or clear.

Associated Symptoms: Fever and malaise are less prevalent in bacterial infections compared to Alaska Pox. Diagnostic Tests:

Bacterial cultures can confirm the particular bacteria, whereas PCR tests detect Alaska Pox.

3. Monkeypox:

Geographic Location: Currently more widespread in particular places, monkeypox warrants assessment based on travel history and prospective exposure.

Lesion Evolution: Monkeypox lesions grow through several stages, commencing flat and evolving to pustules, similar to Alaska Pox.

Lymphadenopathy: Both illnesses induce enlarged lymph nodes, but monkeypox frequently includes more extensive node involvement. Diagnostic testing: PCR testing discriminates between the two viruses with good accuracy.

4. Varicella (Chickenpox):
Vaccination Status: If not vaccinated, varicella can provide a difficulty, especially for elderly adults with diminishing immunity.

Lesion Distribution: Varicella normally spreads broadly over the body, while Alaska Pox tends to cluster.

Lesion Appearance: Varicella lesions are smaller, more frequent, and itchier than Alaska Pox pustules. Diagnostic Testing: Serological testing can detect prior varicella infection, whereas PCR confirms Alaska Pox.

Beyond the Usual Suspects:
Additional problems, including bug bites transmitted by ticks, allergic responses, and unusual skin illnesses, could require care based on individual presentation and travel history. Consulting a healthcare practitioner experienced with Alaska Pox and possible

lookalikes is vital for an appropriate diagnosis.

The Importance of History and Context: Beyond particular symptoms, evaluating your recent activity and probable exposure is key. Sharing facts about travel, outdoor activities, animal interaction, and any known epidemics in your region helps healthcare practitioners make educated evaluations.

Diagnostic Tools: Unveiling the Truth Several methods help in separating Alaska Pox from related illnesses:

Physical inspection: A comprehensive inspection of the skin lesions, noting their location, appearance, and evolution, gives vital insights.

PCR Testing: This extremely sensitive test identifies the virus's genetic material in fluid samples from lesions, enabling a definite diagnosis.

Serological Tests: These tests identify antibodies generated in reaction to the virus but may not be conclusive in the early stages of infection.

Travel History and Exposure Assessment: Evaluating probable ties to known Alaska Pox patients or locations with documented occurrences helps the diagnosis procedure.

Beyond Diagnosis: Supporting Recovery and Future Research

While Alaska Pox still lacks particular therapy, supportive care plays a critical role in facilitating recovery. Ongoing research continues to:

Refine and develop new diagnostic techniques to increase accuracy and speed of diagnosis. Explore possible antiviral medicines to decrease disease duration and minimize consequences.

Investigate the complete range of possible lookalikes and enhance differential diagnostic techniques.

Increase public awareness and education about Alaska Pox and related symptoms to urge early medical intervention. By remaining educated, obtaining expert help, and supporting continuing research, we can traverse the complicated landscape of Alaska Pox symptoms and diagnosis, ensuring informed decisions and successful public health interventions.

Diagnostic tests and procedures

While now offering modest danger, early and exact diagnosis is critical for individual well-being and successful public health initiatives. So, let's begin on a voyage to unravel the subtleties of Alaska Pox diagnosis, covering a number of tests and treatments that help expose the truth.

The Toolbox of Detection: Unveiling Diagnostic Approaches

Several tools play a key role in diagnosing Alaska Pox, and their selection varies depending on individual circumstances and the stage of the illness. Here's a full exploration of each method:

1. The Art of Observation: Physical Examination:

The process begins with a "meticulous physical examination" by a healthcare practitioner. They will carefully assess:

Skin Lesions: Location, size, quantity, appearance (pimples, pustules, ulcers), clustering, distribution, and any evidence of crusting or scarring are painstakingly noted.

Swollen Lymph Nodes: The size, pain, and position of swollen lymph nodes, particularly surrounding the lesions, give crucial insights.

Additional Symptoms: Fever, muscular aches, weariness, and joint discomfort are recorded and assessed in combination with skin findings.

2. Unveiling the Viral Fingerprint Polymerase Chain Reaction (PCR) Test:

This very sensitive test serves as the "gold standard for conclusive diagnosis. A swab sample is obtained from the lesion, and the PCR technique reveals the existence of the Alaska Pox virus's unique genetic material. Results are often available within a few days, enabling rapid and accurate confirmation.

3. Serological Sleuthing: Antibody Testing:

These tests evaluate your blood for antibodies created by your immune system in reaction to the infection. However, they have limitations:

Delayed Detection: Antibodies take time to form, making these tests useful in the early stages of illness.

Previous Exposure vs. Active Illness: Positive findings suggest previous exposure or present infection, necessitating further tests for a final diagnosis.

Distinct types of tests: Two frequent tests, IgM and IgG, give distinct information:

IGM: Detects recent exposure and is often positive 1-2 weeks following the symptom start.

IGG: Indicates prior exposure or long-term illness and stays positive even after recovery.

4. Culture Techniques: Exploring Alternatives:

While less typically employed, viral culture involves cultivating the virus from a lesion sample in a laboratory. This procedure can prove the existence of Alaska Pox, but it takes longer and requires specialist facilities.

5. Travel History and Exposure Assessment:

Understanding your previous actions and probable exposure to the virus is vital. Sharing facts about travel, outdoor excursions, animal interaction, and any known epidemics in your region helps healthcare practitioners make educated judgments regarding additional testing and diagnosis.

Beyond the Basics: Specialized Techniques

In exceptional instances or for research objectives, further procedures could be employed:

Direct Immunofluorescence Assay (DFA): Rapidly detects viral antigens (proteins) in lesion samples, but requires specialized equipment and expertise.

Electron Microscopy: Offers detailed visualization of the virus particles, but is primarily used for research or confirmation in complex cases.

Navigating the Diagnosis Labyrinth:

The best appropriate diagnostic strategy frequently comprises a mix of approaches, considering considerations like:

Stage of infection: PCR is favored for early diagnosis, but serology could be beneficial later.

Severity of symptoms: More comprehensive testing could be necessary for unusual presentations or people with impaired immune systems.

Availability of resources: PCR may be readily available at specialist centers, whereas serological testing could be more accessible in ordinary healthcare settings.

Beyond Diagnosis: Future Directions and Research

Ongoing research activities attempt to:

Refine existing tests: Improve sensitivity, specificity, and speed of diagnostic methods.

Develop new tests: Explore rapid point-of-care tests for faster diagnosis in remote areas.

Standardize diagnostic protocols: Ensure consistent and reliable diagnosis across different healthcare settings. Increase public awareness and education: Empower individuals to recognize potential symptoms and seek early medical attention.

By knowing the present diagnostic methods, respecting their limits, and supporting continuing research, we may traverse the ever-evolving terrain of Alaska Pox diagnosis with educated knowledge and readiness. This permits prompt actions, protecting individual well-being and defending public health from possible dangers.

Chapter 3: Individual Risk and Complications

Factors influencing susceptibility

Alaska Pox opens a new area for studying susceptibility and associated consequences. While currently providing negligible danger to the general population, knowing variables determining individual susceptibility and possible effects of infection strengthens both personal and public health actions. So, let's begin on a voyage to explore the terrain of Alaska Pox risk, navigating elements that may raise exposure and potential consequences related to the virus.

The Susceptibility Spectrum: Unveiling Risk Factors

Our particular vulnerability to Alaska Pox is like a tapestry constructed from diverse threads. While the exact picture remains incomplete, these are important elements that could potentially increase your risk:

1. Exposure Routes:

Direct Contact: Close contact with sick animals, their tissues, or contaminated items offers the biggest danger. This includes acts like handling caught animals, skinning hunting animals, or engaging with ill or deceased wildlife.

Indirect Contact: Environmental contamination with infected animal droppings or secretions can constitute a danger, particularly for people working or spending time outdoors in Alaska.

Aerosols: While the likelihood of airborne transmission requires additional examination, it cannot be fully ruled out, especially in poorly ventilated settings or during close contact with sick animals.

2. Individual Defense System

Immune System Strength: Individuals with impaired immune systems owing to underlying health issues, age, or drug usage could be more susceptible to serious effects upon infection.

Vaccination Status: Currently, no vaccine exists for Alaska Pox. However, research is studying possible vaccine development for greater readiness in the future.

Genetic Predisposition: While research is underway, some genetic variables could impact individual susceptibility or response to the virus.

3. Occupational and Recreational Activities:

Profession: Individuals working in sectors with a higher risk of animal interaction, such as wildlife biologists, veterinarians, or hunters, could have elevated exposure risks.

Outdoor Activities: Engaging in outdoor activities in Alaskan locations with known animal reservoirs enhances the possibility of interactions with sick animals or contaminated settings.

Beyond Susceptibility: Unveiling Potential Complications

While most known Alaska Pox cases have been minor, identifying possible consequences helps patients and healthcare providers handle the virus effectively. However, it's crucial to realize that individual experiences might differ, and difficulties are not assured in every situation.

Potential Complications:

Secondary Bacterial Infections: Skin lesions linked to Alaska Pox can become infected with bacteria, leading to consequences including cellulitis or abscesses. Proper wound care and cleanliness are vital to avoiding these secondary infections.

Swollen Lymph Nodes: While a frequent symptom, swollen lymph nodes can occasionally become painful or irritated, needing special monitoring and therapy.

Long-Term Effects: The long-term implications of the Alaska Pox infection are presently unknown, and further study is needed to determine possible dangers.

Sharing the Responsibility: Public Health Measures
Understanding risk factors and consequences also stresses the necessity of public health initiatives.

Surveillance and Monitoring: Tracking animal populations, human cases, and potential environmental contamination allows for early detection and mitigation of outbreaks.

Public Education and Awareness:
Educating the public about Alaska Pox,
transmission risks, preventive measures,
and the importance of seeking medical
attention empowers individuals to protect
themselves and their communities.

Developing Guidelines and Regulations:
Implementing guidelines for safe handling of
wildlife, proper disposal of animal waste,
and biosecurity measures in research
facilities minimizes potential spillovers from
animals to humans.

**Looking Ahead: The Tapestry Continues
to Unfold**
Ongoing research holds the key to further
understanding the rich fabric of Alaska Pox
susceptibility and consequences. Key areas
of concentration include:

Identifying additional risk factors:
Understanding how various factors interact

to influence susceptibility can inform targeted prevention strategies.

Studying long-term effects: Long-term follow-up of infected individuals helps assess potential complications and guide healthcare management.

Developing antiviral therapies: Exploring potential medications to shorten illness duration and mitigate complications in vulnerable individuals.

Potential complications and high-risk groups

Alaska Pox provides an intriguing scientific curiosity and a possible public health hazard. While now offering negligible danger to the general population, recognizing future problems and identifying high-risk populations strengthens both personal and public health actions. So, let's begin on a tour through the rapids of Alaska Pox, studying the various effects of infection and those most vulnerable to them.

Beyond the Mild: Unveiling Potential Complications

Most known Alaska Pox cases have been minor, appearing with skin lesions and sometimes flu-like symptoms. However, it's vital to note that individual experiences might differ, and any difficulties, though not assured, need attention.

Spectrum of Complications:
1. Secondary Bacterial Infections: Skin lesions, while initially caused by the virus, can become gateways for opportunistic bacteria, leading to illnesses like:

Cellulitis: This painful skin illness involves deeper tissue inflammation and requires antibiotic therapy.

Abscesses: localized collections of pus, typically needing drainage and medication.

2. Disseminated Infection: In rare situations, the virus can travel beyond the primary infection site, impacting internal organs and potentially leading to:

Pneumonia: inflammation of the lungs, presenting with respiratory difficulties.

Encephalitis: inflammation of the brain, causing severe neurological symptoms.

3. Long-Term Effects: While currently unclear, the long-term repercussions of the Alaska Pox infection cannot be fully ruled out. An ongoing study is exploring possible dangers, such as:

Scarring: Skin lesions could heal with persistent scarring, particularly if additional bacterial infections occur. Immunological

Sequelae: The influence on the immune system and possibly increased susceptibility to other infections require more exploration.

Identifying the Vulnerable: High-Risk Groups

While everyone should be aware of Alaska Pox, some people face a heightened risk of consequences because of their innate vulnerability.

1. Individuals with Compromised Immune Systems: Underlying Medical Conditions: People with HIV/AIDS, organ transplant recipients, or those receiving cancer treatment have weaker immune systems, making them more vulnerable to serious infections and consequences.

Age: Infants and elderly individuals often have lower immune systems, increasing their risk.

2. Pregnant Women and Infants: Fetal and Infant Hazards: While evidence on Alaska Pox in pregnant women is sparse, possible hazards to the fetus or baby necessitate strict monitoring and professional care.

Newborn Vulnerability: Young babies have undeveloped immune systems, rendering them more susceptible to serious diseases.

3. Individuals with Skin Diseases Pre-existing Skin Issues: Existing skin diseases such as eczema or dermatitis can aggravate the Alaska Pox infection and raise the likelihood of subsequent bacterial infections.

Beyond Individual Risk: Public Health Responsibility:
Understanding high-risk populations underlines the need for public health initiatives.

1. Targeted Vaccination (if available):
Should a vaccine become available in the future, prioritizing high-risk individuals for immunization would be vital to reducing problems.

2. Enhanced Public Education Tailored awareness efforts targeting high-risk populations, stressing possible dangers, preventative actions, and the significance of obtaining prompt medical assistance are necessary.

3. Surveillance and Early Detection:
Proactive monitoring of high-risk populations and probable exposure scenarios enables early intervention and outbreak management.

Looking Ahead: Charting a Safer Course
Ongoing research holds the key to further understanding Alaska Pox consequences and successfully safeguarding high-risk

individuals. Key areas of concentration include:

Investigating long-term effects:
Long-term follow-up studies involving high-risk populations will give useful insights into potential consequences and inform prevention actions.

Developing antiviral therapies: Exploring drugs particularly targeting Alaska Pox might greatly lower the likelihood of consequences.

Strengthening healthcare infrastructure: ensuring healthcare institutions are able to manage possible epidemics and offer specialized treatment for high-risk groups is critical.

Managing underlying health conditions alongside Alaska Pox

Alaska Pox presents a particular challenge for those with underlying health issues. While currently offering negligible danger to the general public, understanding how underlying diseases could interact with the Alaska Pox infection enables informed decision-making and optimum disease care. So, let's begin on a voyage across this diverse landscape, studying the various problems and techniques for traversing them successfully.

The Intertwined Paths: Understanding Complexities

Individuals with underlying health issues confront a difficult scenario while facing Alaska Pox. Their pre-existing health conditions might impact vulnerability, illness severity, and treatment options. Here's a summary of significant considerations:

1. Weakened Immune Systems:
Many underlying disorders, such as HIV/AIDS, organ transplant recipient status, or continuous cancer therapy, weaken the immune system's capacity to fight infections. This can:

Increase vulnerability to Alaska Pox: Weakened defenses make patients more likely to develop the virus upon exposure.

Prolong and intensify symptoms: The immune system could struggle to manage the virus, resulting in more severe or extended sickness.

Raise the risk of complications: Secondary bacterial infections, disseminated illness, and potential long-term repercussions become more problematic for immunocompromised patients.

2. Specific Conditions and Concerns:

Certain underlying problems demand specific attention:

Respiratory conditions: Asthma or chronic obstructive pulmonary disease (COPD) could be aggravated by Alaska Pox-related respiratory symptoms.

Autoimmune diseases: Lupus or rheumatoid arthritis can interfere with antiviral drugs used to treat Alaska Pox, necessitating cautious monitoring.

Skin conditions: Eczema or dermatitis might enhance susceptibility to subsequent bacterial infections originating from Alaska Pox lesions.

3. Medication Interactions:

Medications used to control underlying diseases could interfere with possible Alaska Pox therapies, necessitating cautious consideration.

Antiviral medicines: Some regularly used antiviral treatments could have contraindications with medications for specific health problems.

Immunosuppressants: Individuals receiving immunosuppressants for situations such as organ transplants could need changes to their drug regimen during an Alaska Pox infection.

Charting a Safe Course: Strategies for Effective Management

Here are crucial ways to handle an Alaska Pox infection with an underlying health condition:

1. Proactive Communication:

Inform your healthcare provider: Immediately discuss any Alaska Pox exposure or symptoms with your doctor, regardless of perceived severity. Share your medical history: Provide a detailed overview of your underlying health condition, medications, and any potential concerns. Maintain open communication: Regularly update your doctor about your symptoms, progress, and any concerns throughout the illness.

2. Tailored Treatment Plans:

Individualized approach: Your doctor will establish a treatment strategy considering your individual health condition, Alaska Pox severity, and any medication interactions. alternate drugs: If traditional antiviral medications entail hazards, seeking alternate treatment options could be essential.

Close monitoring: Regular check-ups and potential revisions to your treatment plan promote effective management and reduce problems.

3. Preventive Measures:
Minimize exposure risk: Follow public health guidelines and avoid situations with high exposure potential, especially if your immune system is significantly compromised.

Practice good hygiene: Frequent handwashing, avoiding close contact with sick individuals, and proper wound care for skin lesions are crucial to preventing secondary infections.

Maintain a healthy lifestyle: Prioritizing healthy nutrition, proper sleep, and stress management enhances your immune system and promotes general well-being.

4. Accessing Support Systems:
Connect with patient advocacy groups: Organizations dedicated to specific health disorders can provide vital information, support, and access to resources.

Seek mental health support: Managing a new illness alongside an existing health condition can be emotionally hard. Consider obtaining professional guidance to handle stress, anxiety, and other emotional difficulties.

Looking Ahead: The Quest for Knowledge Continues

Ongoing research initiatives attempt to further understand the complicated relationships between Alaska Pox and other underlying health issues. Key areas of concentration include:

Investigating specific interactions: Studying how Alaska Pox affects individuals with different health conditions will inform targeted treatment strategies.

Developing safer antiviral medications: Exploring medications with fewer side effects and minimal interactions with existing medications for chronic conditions.

Enhancing public awareness: Educating healthcare providers and the public about controlling Alaska Pox with underlying health issues is critical for optimum care.

Part 2: Living with Alaska Pox

Chapter 4: Treatment and Management Strategies

Current medical approaches and supportive care

Alaska Pox is a distinct medical issue necessitating innovative ways of treatment and management. While currently offering low danger, recognizing the various alternatives empowers consumers and healthcare providers to navigate this unknown environment. So, let's continue on a voyage through the different medicinal methods and supportive care measures for Alaska Pox.

The Treatment Landscape: Available Medical Approaches

Currently, no particular antiviral drug or vaccination is available for Alaska Pox. However, numerous medical treatments are performed to control symptoms and reduce complications.

1. Supportive Care:

Pain Management: Over-the-counter pain medicines such as acetaminophen or ibuprofen can help control discomfort associated with fever, muscular pains, and headaches. In extreme circumstances, stronger pain drugs could be administered.

Wound Care: Maintaining adequate hygiene and washing the skin lesions with mild soap and water helps avoid further bacterial infections. Applying topical creams or dressings could be advised to improve healing and alleviate pain.

Rest and Hydration: Allowing your body appropriate rest and being hydrated with fluids like water are vital for aiding the immune system's battle against the infection.

2. Antiviral Therapies:
While belumravedish has not proved beneficial against Alaska Pox, it could be investigated on a case-by-case basis, particularly for those with severe or persistent illnesses. However, due to its potential adverse effects and lack of clear proof, this strategy requires cautious evaluation by healthcare specialists.

3. Antibiotics:
These are not directly effective against the virus but may be recommended if secondary bacterial infections develop within or around the skin sores.

4. Immunomodulatory Strategies:
In rare situations and based on individual circumstances, healthcare practitioners

could consider utilizing drugs that modify the immune system's response, particularly for those with severe problems or impaired immunity. However, such procedures require continuous supervision and involve significant hazards.

Beyond Medication: The Power of Supportive Care

Supportive care plays a critical role in encouraging healing and well-being alongside any necessary medical measures. Here are crucial elements to consider:

Nutritional Support: Maintaining a balanced diet rich in fruits, vegetables, and whole grains offers critical nutrients to support the immune system and promote healing.

Mental Health Support: Managing a new illness can be stressful, particularly for those with underlying health concerns. Seeking professional mental health care can help

resolve anxiety, stress, and emotional
difficulties.

Patient Education: Empowering yourself
with the correct knowledge of Alaska Pox,
its symptoms, and management techniques
aids in educated decision-making and
encourages self-care.

Connect with Support Groups: Sharing
experiences and connecting with people
experiencing similar situations can provide
emotional support and useful insights.

Looking Ahead: The Evolving Landscape of Treatment

Ongoing research activities attempt to
enhance existing techniques and establish
new ways for controlling Alaska Pox.

**Developing specialized antiviral
medications**: Research is currently
developing antiviral treatments, particularly

targeting Alaska Pox, to provide more focused and effective treatment options.

Investigating immunomodulatory therapies: Further research is needed to understand the possible advantages and hazards of modifying the immune response to an Alaska Pox infection.

Exploring vaccine development: Research efforts are underway to create safe and effective vaccinations that might prevent Alaska Pox infection in the future.

Improving supportive care strategies: Optimizing nutritional and mental health support, along with wound care approaches, will continue to be a focus to increase patient outcomes.

Home care and symptom management

Alaska Pox presents a unique problem necessitating proactive home care and excellent symptom control. While currently offering low danger, recognizing these characteristics helps patients navigate their rehabilitation comfortably and securely. So, let's begin on a trip to investigate techniques for treating Alaska Pox symptoms and supporting recovery within the comfortable shelter of your home.

The Symphony of Symptoms: Recognizing and Managing:
Before getting into home care solutions, let's explore the primary symptoms of Alaska Pox to adapt management approaches:

Skin Lesions: These distinctive features, originally mimicking insect bites, progress into pustules or ulcers. Gentle washing with gentle soap and water, followed by patting dry, is necessary. Avoid severe washing or picking at the lesions, since this might raise the risk of scarring or subsequent infections.

Fever: Manage a moderate fever with over-the-counter drugs such as acetaminophen or ibuprofen. Ensure proper rest and hydration to boost the body's natural defenses.

Muscle pains and joint discomfort: Over-the-counter pain medications could provide assistance. Applying warm compresses to troubled regions and mild stretching might also bring comfort.

Fatigue: Prioritize rest and allow your body adequate time to recoup. Delegate duties and minimize overexertion, favoring sleep and relaxation.

The Home Haven: Creating a Supportive Environment

Turning your house into a refuge for healing entails several critical areas:

1. Hygiene and Isolation:

Frequent handwashing: Rigorous hand hygiene with soap and water, especially after contacting lesions or infected surfaces, is crucial to prevent the transmission of the virus.

Isolate from others: If feasible, maintain physical distance from family members and housemates, particularly young children, pregnant women, or those with impaired immune systems. Dedicate separate towels, cutlery, and linens to decrease transmission risk.

Disinfect surfaces: Regularly clean commonly touched surfaces, including doorknobs, counters, and bathroom fixtures, with proper disinfectants following the manufacturer's directions.

2. Comfort and Relief:

Cool, loose clothing: Wear loose-fitting, breathable clothing to avoid irritating the skin lesions and promote airflow.

Soothing baths: Lukewarm baths with oatmeal or baking soda can help alleviate itching and discomfort associated with the lesions.

Pain management: Stick to recommended dosages of over-the-counter pain relievers prescribed by your doctor. If discomfort persists, visit your healthcare practitioner for more information.

3. Nourishment and Hydration:

Balanced diet: Prioritize a healthy diet rich in fruits, vegetables, and whole grains to provide critical vitamins and minerals that assist your immune system's battle against the virus.

Stay hydrated: Drink lots of fluids like water, herbal teas, or clear broths to maintain hydration and prevent dehydration, especially during fever or sweating.

4. Mental and emotional well-being:
Rest and relaxation: Prioritize enough sleep and relaxation to allow your body to recoup and renew its defenses. Practice relaxing activities like meditation, deep breathing exercises, or light reading to relieve stress and anxiety.

Connect with loved ones: While keeping physical distance, stay connected with friends and family electronically or through phone conversations to battle feelings of loneliness and create emotional support.

Seek professional help: If you are battling with anxiety, despair, or overwhelming emotions, reach out to a mental health professional for guidance and support.

Beyond Home Care: Seeking Professional Guidance

While home care plays a key role, remember that getting professional medical help is necessary in certain situations:

Worsening symptoms: If fever persists, skin lesions become exceedingly painful or spread substantially, or you feel trouble breathing, chest discomfort, or disorientation, seek emergency medical attention.

Underlying health conditions: Individuals with impaired immune systems, pregnant women, and young children require careful monitoring and could benefit from extra guidance from their healthcare professional.

Concerns and inquiries: Don't hesitate to call your doctor if you have any questions or concerns regarding your symptoms, medications, or home care practices.

Navigating the Evolving Landscape: Ongoing research is critical for enhancing home care and symptom control options for Alaska Pox.

Developing rapid diagnostic tests: Faster and more accessible diagnostic tools would enable earlier interventions and targeted home care measures.

Exploring new antiviral medications: Research focusing on specific antiviral therapies for Alaska Pox could potentially shorten illness duration and alleviate symptoms.

Improving symptom management protocols: Studies studying the effectiveness of various complementary treatments and improving pain management procedures might boost patient comfort and recovery.

Addressing psychological and social impacts

Alaska Pox provides not simply a physical challenge but also a possible minefield of psychological and social implications. While currently presenting little danger, understanding and resolving these emotional and interpersonal ramifications is crucial for overall well-being during and after infection. So, let's go on a cruise to examine the secret currents of Alaska Pox, navigating the psychological and sociological nuances it entails.

The Invisible Toll: Unveiling the Psychological Landscape

Alaska Pox may generate a number of emotions, hitting individuals in unique ways. Here are some significant psychological issues to consider:

Anxiety and fear: Uncertainty surrounding the virus, potential complications, and transmission risks can fuel anxiety and fear.

Isolation and loneliness: Physical distancing measures and quarantine protocols can lead to feelings of isolation and loneliness, particularly for individuals living alone or facing limited social contact.

Stigma and discrimination: Misinformation or negative societal perceptions surrounding Alaska Pox can lead to stigmatization and discrimination, further amplifying emotional distress.

Stress and worry: Managing symptoms, potential financial burdens, and disruptions to daily life can create significant stress and worry.

Depression and hopelessness: Prolonged illness, social isolation, and emotional challenges can contribute to feelings of depression and hopelessness.

Seeking Safe Harbor: Strategies for Emotional Well-being

Addressing these psychological repercussions is crucial for successful recovery and long-term well-being. Here are key techniques to handle the emotional terrain:

Seek professional assistance: Don't hesitate to seek out a therapist, counselor, or mental health professional for specific direction and help in managing stress, anxiety, or other emotional concerns.

Practice relaxation techniques:
Techniques like mindfulness meditation,
deep breathing exercises, or yoga can help
manage stress, anxiety, and increase
general well-being.

Engage in wonderful activities: Prioritize
activities you find joyful, whether it's
reading, listening to music, spending time in
nature (where safe), or indulging in hobbies.

Maintain a healthy lifestyle: Prioritize
sleep, eat nutritious meals, and exercise
regularly (as tolerated) to support your
physical and mental health. Join support
groups: Connecting with individuals facing
similar challenges may provide important
insight, empathy, and a feeling of
community.

Beyond the Individual: The Ripple Effect of Social Impacts:
Alaska Pox may also have serious social effects, harming families, communities, and even workplaces.

Disruption of daily life: School closures, workplace shutdowns, and travel restrictions can disrupt daily routines and create logistical challenges.

Financial strain: Medical bills, lost wages due to illness or quarantine, and childcare needs can create financial burdens for individuals and families.

Strain on healthcare systems: Outbreaks can place stress on healthcare systems and resources, requiring effective management strategies.

Misinformation and fear mongering:
Inaccurate information or sensationalized media coverage can fuel fear and hinder public health efforts.

Building Bridges: Fostering Social Support and Solidarity

Addressing these socioeconomic repercussions involves joint action and community-level support:

Accurate and timely information: Public health authorities and media outlets have a responsibility to provide accurate, evidence-based information to combat misinformation and promote informed decision-making.

Social support systems: Strengthening social safety nets and ensuring access to financial assistance for affected individuals and families can mitigate the socioeconomic burdens of Alaska Pox.

Community engagement: Collaborative efforts involving healthcare professionals, community leaders, and the public are crucial for effective outbreak response and social support initiatives.

Combating stigma and discrimination: Educational campaigns promoting understanding and empathy can challenge negative perceptions and prevent social exclusion of individuals affected by Alaska Pox.

Looking Ahead: Navigating the Evolving Landscape

Ongoing research and collaborative actions can expand our understanding and refine strategies for addressing the psychological and social effects of Alaska Pox.

Developing culturally sensitive support: Tailoring support approaches to diverse communities and addressing cultural needs is crucial for ensuring equitable access and effectiveness.

Strengthening communication and collaboration: Fostering open communication and collaboration between researchers, public health officials, and communities is essential for effectively addressing the social and psychological aspects of outbreaks.

Chapter 5: Prevention and Public Health Measures

Individual actions to minimize risk

Alaska Pox poses a new frontier in public health preparation. While currently posing negligible danger to the broader population, recognizing and taking individual preventative steps empowers us to safeguard ourselves and contribute to collective mitigation efforts. So, let's embark on a voyage to investigate the armory of personal measures we may take to limit Alaska Pox risk.

The Armor of Awareness: Individual Preventive Measures:

Now, let's outfit ourselves with specific protective measures, like a robust suit of armor:

1. Minimize contact with potential sources:

Avoid high-risk activities: If possible, refrain from activities with high exposure risk, like handling live animals or visiting areas with known infected animal populations in Alaska.

Practice safe interactions: If necessary interactions occur, wear protective gear like gloves, masks, and long sleeves when handling potentially infected animals or materials.

Dispose of waste properly: Ensure safe disposal of animal waste and materials potentially contaminated with the virus, following recommended guidelines by wildlife authorities.

2. Maintain good hygiene:

Frequent handwashing: Wash your hands thoroughly with soap and water for at least 20 seconds after any potential interaction

with animals, their habitats, or possibly
contaminated items.

Respiratory hygiene: Cover your mouth
and nose with a tissue or your elbow while
coughing or sneezing, and dispose of old
tissues appropriately. Avoid touching your
face: Refrain from touching your eyes, nose,
and mouth with unwashed hands, as this
might encourage virus transmission.

3. Stay informed and vigilant:
Seek information: Stay informed on current
Alaska Pox information from reputable
sources such as public health authorities
and credible news outlets.

Report potential exposure: If you suspect
exposure to possibly contaminated animals
or surroundings, quickly contact your
healthcare professional.

Monitor symptoms: Be alert to potential Alaska Pox symptoms and get medical assistance if you notice any concerns.

4. Vaccination (if available):

Currently, no vaccination exists for Alaska Pox. However, if one becomes available in the future, consider being vaccinated based on individual risk assessments and advice from healthcare specialists.

Beyond Individual Action: The Public Health Shield:

Individual efforts are strong, while public health policies build the framework for larger protection.

Surveillance and Monitoring: Tracking animal populations, human cases, and potential environmental contamination enables early detection and mitigation of outbreaks.

Public Education and Awareness:
Educating the public about Alaska Pox, transmission risks, preventive measures, and the importance of seeking medical attention empowers individuals and fosters collective responsibility.

Developing Guidelines and Regulations:
Implementing guidelines for safe handling of wildlife, proper disposal of animal waste, and biosecurity measures in research facilities minimizes potential spillovers from animals to humans.

Strengthening Healthcare Systems:
Ensuring healthcare facilities are equipped to manage potential outbreaks and provide optimal care for infected individuals is crucial.

Looking Ahead: Forging a Path of Preparedness

Ongoing research and collaborative activities hold the key to significantly improving our collective protection against Alaska Pox:

Deloping diagnostic tools: Faster and more accessible diagnostic tests would enable earlier interventions and improve public health management.

Exploring antiviral therapies: Investigating potential medications specifically targeting Alaska Pox could mitigate complications and shorten illness duration.

Investing in research and development: Continued research efforts are necessary to understand the virus better, create vaccines, and enhance preventative and therapeutic techniques.

Role of public health agencies and healthcare providers

Alaska Pox presents a distinct challenge, necessitating a concerted response from public health organizations and healthcare practitioners. While currently posing a modest risk, their proactive and coordinated actions are vital for maintaining public health through prevention, early identification, and effective management. Let's look into the exact responsibilities these entities play in constructing a solid line of protection against Alaska Pox.

Public Health Agencies: Guardians of Community Well-Being: Public health authorities operate as the sentinels of community health, employing numerous weapons to battle possible Alaska Pox outbreaks:

1. Surveillance and Monitoring: Leading the charge Public health agencies pioneer animal and human surveillance programs, employing tactics including wildlife population monitoring, testing sentinel animals, and tracking human cases to identify possible outbreaks early.

Data analysis and reporting: They evaluate gathered data, detect patterns, and swiftly report suspected or verified cases to relevant authorities and the public.

Guiding public health interventions: Based on their analysis, they plan and execute evidence-based community-level interventions such as public awareness campaigns, risk reduction measures, and resource allocation.

2. Public Education and Risk Communication

Creating clear and simple information:
Public health organizations are responsible for communicating accurate and accessible information about Alaska Pox, its symptoms, transmission risks, preventative strategies, and available services.

Tailoring communication: They customize communications to varied audiences, considering cultural sensitivities and engaging trusted community leaders to guarantee information reaches all demographics successfully.

Combating disinformation: They aggressively challenge misconceptions and myths concerning Alaska Pox, supporting appropriate conduct and minimizing unwarranted fear mongering.

3. Outbreak Response and Coordination: Leading the response

Public health agencies coordinate and lead epidemic response operations, mobilizing resources, deploying staff, and applying established protocols to control and manage outbreaks efficiently.

Contact tracing and isolation: They identify and track close contacts of infected individuals, advising on isolation and quarantine measures to prevent further transmission.

Supporting healthcare providers: They provide guidance, training, and resources to healthcare providers on Alaska Pox diagnosis, management, and reporting procedures.

4. Policy Development and Enforcement:
Developing regulations: Public health agencies draft and implement regulations related to wildlife management, biosecurity

in research facilities, and proper waste disposal to minimize exposure risks.

Healthcare Providers: Frontline Defenders in Patient Care:

Healthcare practitioners have a vital role in recognizing, diagnosing, and controlling Alaska Pox cases, preserving individual and community health:

1. Early Detection and Diagnosis: Raising awareness

Healthcare practitioners educate patients about Alaska Pox symptoms and advise them to seek medical assistance quickly if worried about exposure or probable infection.

Clinical assessment: They do detailed clinical examinations, evaluating patient history, travel information, and potential exposure risks while examining for distinctive symptoms.

Diagnostic testing: Healthcare practitioners employ available diagnostic tests, following established standards to confirm or rule out Alaska Pox infection.

2. Patient Management and Treatment: Providing supportive care:

They manage symptoms through pain relief, hydration, and wound care, ensuring optimal patient comfort and recovery.

Monitoring and follow-up: Healthcare providers closely monitor patients, assess their progress, and provide necessary follow-up care, including isolation or quarantine recommendations.

3. Community Education and Engagement: Providing accurate information

Healthcare providers play a crucial role in educating their patients and communities about Alaska Pox, addressing concerns, and dispelling misinformation.

Promoting preventive measures: They advocate for individual actions like safe wildlife interaction practices, good hygiene, and seeking medical attention when necessary.

Building trust and confidence: Healthcare practitioners promote trust and confidence within their communities, increasing adherence to public health recommendations and facilitating successful epidemic response.

Chapter 6: Research and Future Outlook

Vaccine development and future prevention strategies

Alaska Pox stands as a sentinel of unknown origin, providing a challenge to both scientific knowledge and public health preparation. While now posing modest risk, the threat of future outbreaks highlights the essential need for comprehensive preventative efforts, notably the development of a safe and efficient vaccine. This chapter digs into the continuing research activities regarding Alaska Pox vaccine development and analyzes the many routes being taken to avert future virus threats.

The Vaccine Imperative:
The absence of a modern vaccination leaves us exposed to prospective Alaska Pox outbreaks. However, the scientific community is currently engaged in a multi-pronged strategy to providing protection:

1. Unveiling the Viral Target:
Antigen identification: Identifying essential viral proteins that generate a protective immune response is critical for vaccine creation. Researchers are painstakingly studying the Alaska Pox genome to discover antigens that trigger powerful neutralizing antibodies or T-cell responses.

Structural studies: Examining the three-dimensional structure of these antigens enables for the construction of vaccinations that replicate their form, causing the immune system to detect and destroy the actual virus. This includes sophisticated methods like X-ray crystallography and cryo-electron microscopy.

2. Exploring Diverse Vaccine Platforms: Live-attenuated vaccines: Weakened variants of the virus that activate the immune system without producing severe sickness have proven useful for different ailments. However, worries regarding potential return to virulence urge cautious study for Alaska Pox.

Subunit vaccines: These vaccines employ only select viral proteins instead of the full virus, enabling greater safety and convenience of manufacture. Identifying immunogenic components and creating effective delivery mechanisms are significant research areas.

Viral vector vaccines: Engineered viruses bearing Alaska Pox antigen genes can transfer them into human cells, causing an immunological response. Exploring safe and effective viral vectors like adenoviruses or measles viruses is ongoing.

DNA vaccines: Plasmid DNA encoding Alaska Pox antigens can be injected into muscle cells, instructing them to produce these antigens and trigger immunity. Optimizing DNA delivery methods and ensuring robust immune responses are research priorities.

3. Bridging the Gap: Preclinical and Clinical Trials:

Animal models: Establishing reliable animal models that mimic human Alaska Pox infection is crucial for testing vaccine candidates before clinical trials. Identifying suitable animal species and ensuring model fidelity are active research areas.

Preclinical testing: Promising vaccine candidates undergo rigorous preclinical studies in animals to assess safety, immunogenicity, and efficacy. These studies provide vital data for informing clinical trial design.

Clinical trials: Once deemed safe and promising in preclinical studies, candidate vaccines progress to carefully controlled clinical trials in humans. Phase I trials assess safety and dosage, while Phase II evaluates efficacy and immune response, and Phase III confirms effectiveness in larger populations.

Beyond the Vaccine: A Multifaceted Approach:
While vaccine development remains central, other promising avenues hold significance in future prevention strategies:

Antiviral medications: Identifying and developing drugs that specifically target Alaska Pox replication are crucial for mitigating disease severity and potentially reducing transmission. Repurposing existing antiviral drugs and exploring novel compounds are active research areas.

Post-exposure prophylaxis: Exploring the potential of administering antiviral medications or immune-boosting agents shortly after potential exposure to Alaska Pox could prevent infection or lessen its severity.

Community-level interventions: Public health measures like promoting good hygiene, responsible wildlife interaction practices, and early medical attention in case of suspected exposure remain crucial for preventing transmission and mitigating outbreaks.

The Horizon Unfurls: Opportunities
Despite these challenges, the future holds opportunities:

Technological advancements: Advances in fields like genomics, immunology, and vaccine delivery systems are creating new possibilities for faster and more effective vaccine development.

Global collaboration: International partnerships between researchers, public health agencies, and governments can accelerate progress, share resources, and ensure equitable access to prevention tools.

Community engagement: Building trust and fostering community participation in research and public health initiatives are crucial for successful implementation of prevention strategies.

Living with Alaska Pox in the long term

Alaska Pox poses not merely a scientific challenge but a potential reality we would have to learn to live with. Adjusting to a world where Alaska Pox persists is vital for individual and community well-being.

Adapting to the New Normal: Strategies for Living with Alaska Pox

While the future remains unpredictable, proactive efforts can strengthen our resilience and ability to adapt:

1. Individual Preparedness:

Stay informed: Remain updated on Alaska Pox developments through reliable sources like public health agencies and credible media outlets.

Practice preventive measures: Maintain good hygiene, avoid risky wildlife interactions, and seek medical attention promptly if concerned about potential exposure.

Prepare for disruptions: Develop contingency plans for potential disruptions to work, travel, or daily life due to outbreaks. Prioritize mental well-being: Practice stress management techniques, seek social support, and access mental health resources if needed.

3. Scientific Innovation:
 Continued research: Ongoing study into Alaska Pox biology, diagnostics, treatments, and vaccinations is vital for creating long-term solutions. Exploring emerging technologies: Investigate creative ways like gene editing or mRNA vaccines for possible future interventions.

One Health approach: Recognize the connection of animal and human health, fostering collaborative research and solutions across disciplines.

4. Mental Health and Well-being: Promote mental health awareness: Normalize seeking help for stress, anxiety, or other mental health challenges arising from living with Alaska Pox.

Increase access to mental health services: Expand access to mental health professionals and culturally appropriate support systems within communities.

Part 3: Conclusion

Additional resources and organizations

Living with the potential threat of Alaska Pox necessitates staying informed and accessing reliable resources. This appendix provides a curated list of valuable resources and organizations dedicated to Alaska Pox research, public health response, and individual preparedness. Remember, consulting qualified healthcare professionals and official public health agencies remains crucial for obtaining specific guidance and recommendations.

Government Agencies
Centers for Disease Control and Prevention (CDC): Provides up-to-date information on Alaska Pox, including symptoms, transmission, prevention, and outbreak updates.

World Health Organization (WHO): Offers global perspectives on emerging infectious diseases like Alaska Pox, including technical resources and outbreak response guidance.

National Institutes of Health (NIH): Supports research on Alaska Pox through various institutes, including the National Institute of Allergy and Infectious Diseases (NIAID).

Alaska Department of Health and Social Services (DHSS): Provides Alaska-specific information on Alaska Pox, including surveillance data, public health recommendations, and local resources.

Scientific Resources
National Library of Medicine (NLM): Offers access to scientific publications and databases relevant to Alaska Pox research, including PubMed and MEDLINE.
ScienceDirect
World Organisation for Animal Health (OIE):

Non-Governmental Organizations (NGOs):
Global Health Organization (GHO):
Médecins Sans Frontières (MSF):
Project ECHO

Myth busters: Addressing common misconceptions and misinformation

In an age of plentiful information, distinguishing reality from fiction around rising health hazards like Alaska Pox may be tough. This appendix debunks common myths and disinformation spreading about the virus, providing you with factual knowledge to protect yourself and your community.

Myth 1: Alaska Pox is the same as smallpox.

Fact: While both viruses belong to the Orthopoxvirus genus, they are independent organisms with distinctive properties. Smallpox was eliminated globally in 1980, but Alaska Pox is a unique virus with continuing study to comprehend its complete clinical spectrum and severity.

Myth 2: Alaska Pox is very infectious and readily spreads between people.

Fact: The present understanding shows Alaska Pox could have minimal human-to-human transmission, while additional work is continuing. Most documented occurrences involve direct contact with diseased animals or contaminated items.

Myth 3: There is no vaccination or cure for Alaska Pox.

Fact: While no licensed vaccination or particular therapy presently exists, research efforts are actively ongoing to produce both. Public health interventions, including excellent cleanliness and avoiding dangerous animal contacts, remain critical for prevention.

Myth 4: The risk of Alaska Pox is overblown, and there's no reason to worry.

Fact: While the present danger might be modest, identifying and planning for potential future hazards is crucial. Public health officials regularly monitor the situation and give advice based on new knowledge

Myth 5: Consuming particular meals or supplements will prevent Alaska Pox infection.

Fact: There is no scientific evidence to back claims that any one meal or supplement gives protection against Alaska Pox. Focusing on preventative measures advised by public health authorities remains the most effective method.

Myth 6: Only persons who travel to Alaska are in danger of developing Alaska Pox.

Fact: While the initial cases were detected in Alaska, the potential for the virus to spread to other locations exists. Staying updated about the newest advances and following public health advice regardless of region is vital.

Myth 7: Wearing a mask can protect you from breathing the Alaska Pox virus.
Fact: The present knowledge shows the principal transmission mechanism might not be airborne. However, adopting normal respiratory hygiene measures like wearing masks in crowded places or while having respiratory symptoms is always suggested.

Myth 8: Only persons with severe symptoms need to seek medical assistance for probable Alaska Pox exposure.
Fact: Even if you experience minor symptoms or suspect probable exposure, rapidly seeking medical assistance is vital for early diagnosis, isolation if necessary, and contributing to public health efforts.

Myth 9: There is a government cover-up over the real severity of the Alaska Pox outbreak.

Fact: Public health authorities and organizations like the CDC and WHO promote transparency and give regular updates based on current scientific knowledge. Trusting official sources and avoiding spreading disinformation is crucial.

Myth 10: Stockpiling drugs or supplies is vital to prepare for an Alaska Pox outbreak.

Fact: Following public health suggestions, including maintaining excellent cleanliness, avoiding dangerous animal contacts, and getting medical assistance when required, is the most effective approach to preparing. Excessive hoarding can generate needless shortages and limit access for people who actually need them.

9 798887 968583 1